My Mood Journal

A record of how what I eat, moon cycles, and more affect my mood.

Designed by Cheryl Roby

Copyright 2014 Cheryl Roby all rights reserved

Cover photo and design by Cheryl Roby

ISBN-13: 978-1494836887

ISBN-10: 1494836882

All rights reserved

Using This Journal

As an Energy Medicine practitioner and a true believer in the mind/body connection, I have long wondered about the relationships between the many factors that affect our wellbeing. This Mood Journal is the outcome of those musings. I designed it to keep track of the phases of the moon, how you sleep, whether you exercise, what you eat, how you feel and more--all in one place. There is also room for daily creative expression through writing and or doodling if you find it helpful. You may want to keep track of other things in the journaling space such as whether you meditated or engaged in any other activity you believe influences how you feel

There are 120 journaling pages herein—enough to track two lunar cycles. By then (or even before) you may be able to spot trends. Are you sleepy or more alert around the time of the full or new moon? What foods energize you? Where were you when you felt the best? The worst?

What you record in these pages will reflect your unique nature. Everything is optional and intended for your benefit. Make modifications to the pages to suit your needs. If you find something particularly helpful, feel free to email me, so I can share it in subsequent versions of this journal.

I hope this journal will help you discover how to feel your very best and how to care for yourself when you are not.

In wellness and gratitude,

Cheryl Roby
www.cherylroby.com
www.robychart.com
email: cheryl@robychart.com

My Mood

Journal

A record of how what I eat, moon cycles, and more affect my mood.

From: _____

To: _____

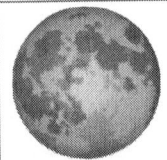 Phase of the moon

New   Waxing   Waning   Full

Date:

How I slept:

What I Ate:
   Morning
   _____
   _____
   _____

   Afternoon
   _____
   _____
   _____

   Evening
   _____
   _____
   _____

How I felt:

   Morning:
   Great/energized
   Neutral/balanced
   Sad/low energy

   Afternoon:
   Great/energized
   Neutral/balanced
   Sad/low energy

   Evening:
   Great/energized
   Neutral/balanced
   Sad/low energy

How much/what type of exercise?

Personal Journal space

Doodle space

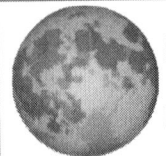 Phase of the moon

New   Waxing   Waning   Full

Date:

How I slept:

What I Ate:
  Morning

  Afternoon

  Evening

How I felt:
  Morning:
    Great/energized
    Neutral/balanced
    Sad/low energy

  Afternoon:
    Great/energized
    Neutral/balanced
    Sad/low energy

  Evening:
    Great/energized
    Neutral/balanced
    Sad/low energy

How much/what type of exercise?

Personal Journal space

Doodle space

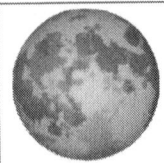 Phase of the moon

New   Waxing   Waning   Full

Date:

How I slept:

What I Ate:
  Morning

How I felt:
  Morning:
  Great/energized
  Neutral/balanced
  Sad/low energy

  Afternoon

  Afternoon:
  Great/energized
  Neutral/balanced
  Sad/low energy

  Evening

  Evening:
  Great/energized
  Neutral/balanced
  Sad/low energy

How much/what type of exercise?

Personal Journal space

Doodle space

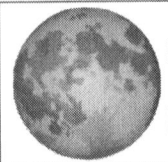

Phase of the moon

New   Waxing   Waning   Full

Date:

How I slept:

What I Ate:

Morning

_____
_____
_____

Afternoon

_____
_____
_____

Evening

_____
_____
_____

How I felt:

Morning:

Great/energized

Neutral/balanced

Sad/low energy

Afternoon:

Great/energized

Neutral/balanced

Sad/low energy

Evening:

Great/energized

Neutral/balanced

Sad/low energy

How much/what type of exercise?

Personal Journal space

Doodle space

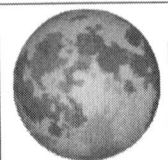 Phase of the moon

New   Waxing   Waning   Full

Date:

How I slept:

What I Ate:
  Morning

_____
_____
_____
_____

  Afternoon

_____
_____
_____
_____

  Evening

_____
_____
_____
_____

How I felt:

  Morning:

  Great/energized

  Neutral/balanced

  Sad/low energy

  Afternoon:

  Great/energized

  Neutral/balanced

  Sad/low energy

  Evening:

  Great/energized

  Neutral/balanced

  Sad/low energy

How much/what type of exercise?

Personal Journal space

Doodle space

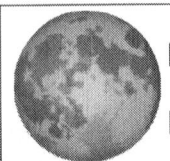

Phase of the moon

New   Waxing   Waning   Full

Date:

How I slept:

What I Ate:

Morning

_____
_____
_____

Afternoon

_____
_____
_____

Evening

_____
_____
_____

How I felt:

Morning:

Great/energized

Neutral/balanced

Sad/low energy

Afternoon:

Great/energized

Neutral/balanced

Sad/low energy

Evening:

Great/energized

Neutral/balanced

Sad/low energy

How much/what type of exercise?

Personal Journal space

Doodle space

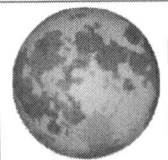

Phase of the moon

New   Waxing   Waning   Full

Date:

How I slept:

What I Ate:
  Morning

  _____
  _____
  _____

  Afternoon

  _____
  _____
  _____

  Evening

  _____
  _____
  _____

How I felt:

  Morning:

  Great/energized

  Neutral/balanced

  Sad/low energy

  Afternoon:

  Great/energized

  Neutral/balanced

  Sad/low energy

  Evening:

  Great/energized

  Neutral/balanced

  Sad/low energy

How much/what type of exercise?

Personal Journal space

Doodle space

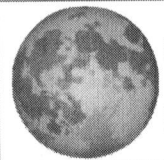 Phase of the moon

New   Waxing   Waning   Full

Date:

How I slept:

What I Ate:
   Morning

_____
_____
_____

   Afternoon

_____
_____
_____

   Evening

_____
_____
_____

How I felt:
   Morning:

   Great/energized

   Neutral/balanced

   Sad/low energy

   Afternoon:

   Great/energized

   Neutral/balanced

   Sad/low energy

   Evening:

   Great/energized

   Neutral/balanced

   Sad/low energy

How much/what type of exercise?

Personal Journal space

Doodle space

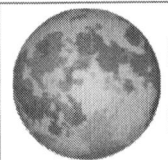

Phase of the moon

New   Waxing   Waning   Full

Date:

How I slept:

What I Ate:

Morning

_____
_____
_____

Afternoon

_____
_____
_____

Evening

_____
_____
_____

How I felt:

Morning:

Great/energized

Neutral/balanced

Sad/low energy

Afternoon:

Great/energized

Neutral/balanced

Sad/low energy

Evening:

Great/energized

Neutral/balanced

Sad/low energy

How much/what type of exercise?

Personal Journal space

Doodle space

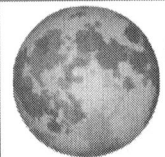 Phase of the moon

New   Waxing   Waning   Full

Date:

How I slept:

What I Ate:
   Morning

   _____
   _____
   _____

   Afternoon

   _____
   _____
   _____

   Evening

   _____
   _____
   _____

How I felt:

   Morning:

   Great/energized

   Neutral/balanced

   Sad/low energy

   Afternoon:

   Great/energized

   Neutral/balanced

   Sad/low energy

   Evening:

   Great/energized

   Neutral/balanced

   Sad/low energy

How much/what type of exercise?

Personal Journal space

Doodle space

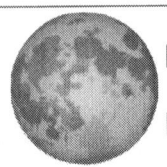

Phase of the moon

New   Waxing   Waning   Full

Date:

How I slept:

What I Ate:

Morning

_____

_____

_____

Afternoon

_____

_____

_____

Evening

_____

_____

_____

How I felt:

Morning:

Great/energized

Neutral/balanced

Sad/low energy

Afternoon:

Great/energized

Neutral/balanced

Sad/low energy

Evening:

Great/energized

Neutral/balanced

Sad/low energy

How much/what type of exercise?

Personal Journal space

Doodle space

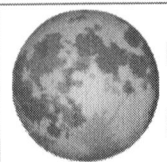 Phase of the moon

New   Waxing   Waning   Full

Date:

How I slept:

What I Ate:
   Morning

_____

_____

_____

   Afternoon

_____

_____

_____

   Evening

_____

_____

_____

How I felt:
   Morning:
      Great/energized
      Neutral/balanced
      Sad/low energy

   Afternoon:
      Great/energized
      Neutral/balanced
      Sad/low energy

   Evening:
      Great/energized
      Neutral/balanced
      Sad/low energy

How much/what type of exercise?

Personal Journal space

Doodle space

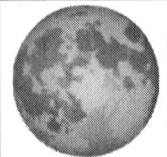 Phase of the moon

New   Waxing   Waning   Full

Date:

How I slept:

What I Ate:
  Morning
  _____
  _____
  _____

  Afternoon
  _____
  _____
  _____

  Evening
  _____
  _____
  _____

How I felt:
  Morning:
  Great/energized
  Neutral/balanced
  Sad/low energy

  Afternoon:
  Great/energized
  Neutral/balanced
  Sad/low energy

  Evening:
  Great/energized
  Neutral/balanced
  Sad/low energy

How much/what type of exercise?

Personal Journal space

Doodle space

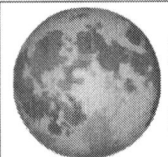 Phase of the moon

New   Waxing   Waning   Full

Date:

How I slept:

What I Ate:

Morning

_____
_____
_____

Afternoon

_____
_____
_____

Evening

_____
_____
_____

How I felt:

Morning:

Great/energized

Neutral/balanced

Sad/low energy

Afternoon:

Great/energized

Neutral/balanced

Sad/low energy

Evening:

Great/energized

Neutral/balanced

Sad/low energy

How much/what type of exercise?

Personal Journal space

Doodle space

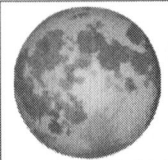

Phase of the moon

New   Waxing   Waning   Full

Date:

How I slept:

What I Ate:

Morning

_____
_____
_____

Afternoon

_____
_____
_____

Evening

_____
_____
_____

How I felt:

Morning:

Great/energized

Neutral/balanced

Sad/low energy

Afternoon:

Great/energized

Neutral/balanced

Sad/low energy

Evening:

Great/energized

Neutral/balanced

Sad/low energy

How much/what type of exercise?

Personal Journal space

Doodle space

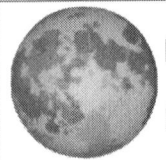

Phase of the moon

New   Waxing   Waning   Full

Date:

How I slept:

What I Ate:

Morning

_____
_____
_____

Afternoon

_____
_____
_____

Evening

_____
_____
_____

How I felt:

Morning:

Great/energized

Neutral/balanced

Sad/low energy

Afternoon:

Great/energized

Neutral/balanced

Sad/low energy

Evening:

Great/energized

Neutral/balanced

Sad/low energy

How much/what type of exercise?

Personal Journal space

Doodle space

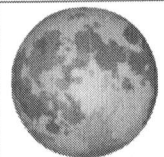

Phase of the moon

New   Waxing   Waning   Full

Date:

How I slept:

What I Ate:
Morning

_____
_____
_____

Afternoon

_____
_____
_____

Evening

_____
_____
_____

How I felt:

Morning:

Great/energized

Neutral/balanced

Sad/low energy

Afternoon:

Great/energized

Neutral/balanced

Sad/low energy

Evening:

Great/energized

Neutral/balanced

Sad/low energy

How much/what type of exercise?

Personal Journal space

Doodle space

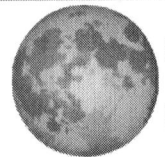

Phase of the moon

New   Waxing   Waning   Full

Date:

How I slept:

What I Ate:

Morning

_____
_____
_____

Afternoon

_____
_____
_____

Evening

_____
_____
_____

How I felt:

Morning:

Great/energized

Neutral/balanced

Sad/low energy

Afternoon:

Great/energized

Neutral/balanced

Sad/low energy

Evening:

Great/energized

Neutral/balanced

Sad/low energy

How much/what type of exercise?

Personal Journal space

Doodle space

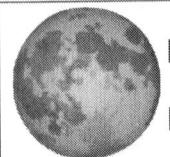

Phase of the moon

New   Waxing   Waning   Full

Date:

How I slept:

What I Ate:
   Morning

How I felt:
   Morning:
   Great/energized
   Neutral/balanced
   Sad/low energy

   Afternoon

   Afternoon:
   Great/energized
   Neutral/balanced
   Sad/low energy

   Evening

   Evening:
   Great/energized
   Neutral/balanced
   Sad/low energy

How much/what type of exercise?

Personal Journal space

Doodle space

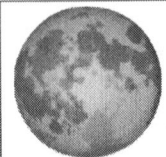

Phase of the moon

New   Waxing   Waning   Full

Date:

How I slept:

What I Ate:

Morning

_____
_____
_____

Afternoon

_____
_____
_____

Evening

_____
_____
_____

How I felt:

Morning:

Great/energized

Neutral/balanced

Sad/low energy

Afternoon:

Great/energized

Neutral/balanced

Sad/low energy

Evening:

Great/energized

Neutral/balanced

Sad/low energy

How much/what type of exercise?

Personal Journal space

Doodle space

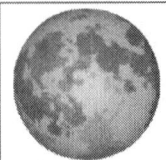

Phase of the moon

New   Waxing   Waning   Full

Date:

How I slept:

What I Ate:

Morning

_____
_____
_____

Afternoon

_____
_____
_____

Evening

_____
_____
_____

How much/what type of exercise?

How I felt:

Morning:

Great/energized

Neutral/balanced

Sad/low energy

Afternoon:

Great/energized

Neutral/balanced

Sad/low energy

Evening:

Great/energized

Neutral/balanced

Sad/low energy

Personal Journal space

Doodle space

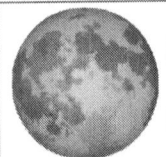

Phase of the moon

New   Waxing   Waning   Full

Date:

How I slept:

What I Ate:
  Morning
  _____
  _____
  _____

  Afternoon
  _____
  _____
  _____

  Evening
  _____
  _____
  _____

How I felt:
  Morning:
    Great/energized
    Neutral/balanced
    Sad/low energy

  Afternoon:
    Great/energized
    Neutral/balanced
    Sad/low energy

  Evening:
    Great/energized
    Neutral/balanced
    Sad/low energy

How much/what type of exercise?

Personal Journal space

Doodle space

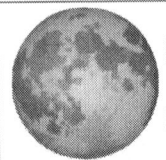

Phase of the moon

New   Waxing   Waning   Full

Date:

How I slept:

What I Ate:
 Morning
 _____
 _____
 _____
 _____

 Afternoon
 _____
 _____
 _____
 _____

 Evening
 _____
 _____
 _____
 _____

How I felt:
 Morning:
  Great/energized
  Neutral/balanced
  Sad/low energy

 Afternoon:
  Great/energized
  Neutral/balanced
  Sad/low energy

 Evening:
  Great/energized
  Neutral/balanced
  Sad/low energy

How much/what type of exercise?

Personal Journal space

Doodle space

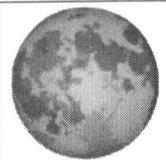

Phase of the moon

New   Waxing   Waning   Full

Date:

How I slept:

What I Ate:
 Morning

Afternoon

Evening

How I felt:
 Morning:
   Great/energized
   Neutral/balanced
   Sad/low energy

 Afternoon:
   Great/energized
   Neutral/balanced
   Sad/low energy

 Evening:
   Great/energized
   Neutral/balanced
   Sad/low energy

How much/what type of exercise?

Personal Journal space

Doodle space

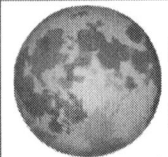

Phase of the moon

New   Waxing   Waning   Full

Date:

How I slept:

What I Ate:
  Morning
  _____
  _____
  _____

  Afternoon
  _____
  _____
  _____

  Evening
  _____
  _____
  _____

How I felt:
  Morning:
  Great/energized
  Neutral/balanced
  Sad/low energy

  Afternoon:
  Great/energized
  Neutral/balanced
  Sad/low energy

  Evening:
  Great/energized
  Neutral/balanced
  Sad/low energy

How much/what type of exercise?

Personal Journal space

Doodle space

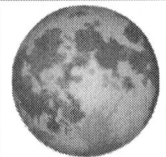 Phase of the moon

New   Waxing   Waning   Full

Date:

How I slept:

What I Ate:

Morning

_____
_____
_____

Afternoon

_____
_____
_____

Evening

_____
_____
_____

How I felt:

Morning:

Great/energized

Neutral/balanced

Sad/low energy

Afternoon:

Great/energized

Neutral/balanced

Sad/low energy

Evening:

Great/energized

Neutral/balanced

Sad/low energy

How much/what type of exercise?

Personal Journal space

Doodle space

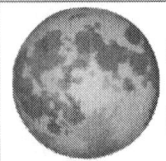 Phase of the moon New Waxing Waning Full	Date:

How I slept:

What I Ate:

Morning

_____
_____
_____

Afternoon

_____
_____
_____

Evening

_____
_____
_____

How I felt:

Morning:

Great/energized

Neutral/balanced

Sad/low energy

Afternoon:

Great/energized

Neutral/balanced

Sad/low energy

Evening:

Great/energized

Neutral/balanced

Sad/low energy

How much/what type of exercise?

Personal Journal space

Doodle space

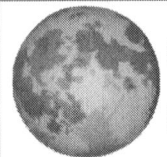

Phase of the moon

New   Waxing   Waning   Full

Date:

How I slept:

What I Ate:

Morning

_____
_____
_____

Afternoon

_____
_____
_____

Evening

_____
_____
_____

How I felt:

Morning:

Great/energized

Neutral/balanced

Sad/low energy

Afternoon:

Great/energized

Neutral/balanced

Sad/low energy

Evening:

Great/energized

Neutral/balanced

Sad/low energy

How much/what type of exercise?

Personal Journal space

Doodle space

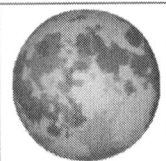

Phase of the moon

New   Waxing   Waning   Full

Date:

How I slept:

What I Ate:

Morning

_____
_____
_____

Afternoon

_____
_____
_____

Evening

_____
_____
_____

How I felt:

Morning:

Great/energized

Neutral/balanced

Sad/low energy

Afternoon:

Great/energized

Neutral/balanced

Sad/low energy

Evening:

Great/energized

Neutral/balanced

Sad/low energy

How much/what type of exercise?

Personal Journal space

Doodle space

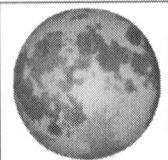 Phase of the moon

New   Waxing   Waning   Full

Date:

How I slept:

What I Ate:
   Morning
   _____
   _____
   _____

   Afternoon
   _____
   _____
   _____

   Evening
   _____
   _____
   _____

How I felt:
   Morning:
   Great/energized
   Neutral/balanced
   Sad/low energy

   Afternoon:
   Great/energized
   Neutral/balanced
   Sad/low energy

   Evening:
   Great/energized
   Neutral/balanced
   Sad/low energy

How much/what type of exercise?

Personal Journal space

Doodle space

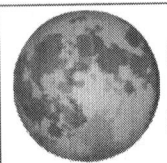 Phase of the moon

New   Waxing   Waning   Full

Date:

How I slept:

What I Ate:
Morning

_____
_____
_____

Afternoon

_____
_____
_____

Evening

_____
_____
_____

How I felt:

Morning:

Great/energized

Neutral/balanced

Sad/low energy

Afternoon:

Great/energized

Neutral/balanced

Sad/low energy

Evening:

Great/energized

Neutral/balanced

Sad/low energy

How much/what type of exercise?

Personal Journal space

Doodle space

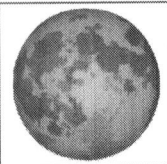 Phase of the moon

New   Waxing   Waning   Full

Date:

How I slept:

What I Ate:
  Morning
  _____
  _____
  _____
  _____

  Afternoon
  _____
  _____
  _____
  _____

  Evening
  _____
  _____
  _____
  _____

How I felt:
  Morning:
  Great/energized
  Neutral/balanced
  Sad/low energy

  Afternoon:
  Great/energized
  Neutral/balanced
  Sad/low energy

  Evening:
  Great/energized
  Neutral/balanced
  Sad/low energy

How much/what type of exercise?

Personal Journal space

Doodle space

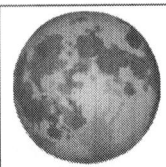 Phase of the moon

New   Waxing   Waning   Full

Date:

How I slept:

What I Ate:
  Morning

  _____
  _____
  _____

  Afternoon

  _____
  _____
  _____

  Evening

  _____
  _____
  _____

How I felt:
  Morning:
    Great/energized
    Neutral/balanced
    Sad/low energy

  Afternoon:
    Great/energized
    Neutral/balanced
    Sad/low energy

  Evening:
    Great/energized
    Neutral/balanced
    Sad/low energy

How much/what type of exercise?

Personal Journal space

Doodle space

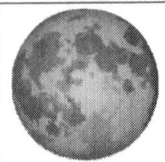

Phase of the moon

New   Waxing   Waning   Full

Date:

How I slept:

What I Ate:
 Morning

_____
_____
_____

 Afternoon

_____
_____
_____

 Evening

_____
_____
_____

How I felt:

 Morning:
  Great/energized
  Neutral/balanced
  Sad/low energy

 Afternoon:
  Great/energized
  Neutral/balanced
  Sad/low energy

 Evening:
  Great/energized
  Neutral/balanced
  Sad/low energy

How much/what type of exercise?

Personal Journal space

Doodle space

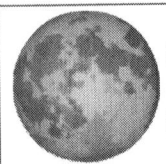

Phase of the moon

New   Waxing   Waning   Full

Date:

How I slept:

What I Ate:

Morning

_____
_____
_____

Afternoon

_____
_____
_____

Evening

_____
_____
_____

How I felt:

Morning:

Great/energized

Neutral/balanced

Sad/low energy

Afternoon:

Great/energized

Neutral/balanced

Sad/low energy

Evening:

Great/energized

Neutral/balanced

Sad/low energy

How much/what type of exercise?

Personal Journal space

Doodle space

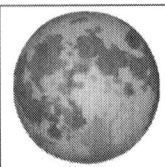 Phase of the moon

New   Waxing   Waning   Full

Date:

How I slept:

What I Ate:
   Morning
   _____
   _____
   _____
   _____

   Afternoon
   _____
   _____
   _____
   _____

   Evening
   _____
   _____
   _____
   _____

How I felt:
   Morning:
      Great/energized
      Neutral/balanced
      Sad/low energy

   Afternoon:
      Great/energized
      Neutral/balanced
      Sad/low energy

   Evening:
      Great/energized
      Neutral/balanced
      Sad/low energy

How much/what type of exercise?

Personal Journal space

Doodle space

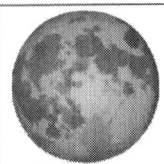

Phase of the moon

New   Waxing   Waning   Full

Date:

How I slept:

What I Ate:

Morning

_____
_____
_____

Afternoon

_____
_____
_____

Evening

_____
_____
_____

How I felt:

Morning:

Great/energized

Neutral/balanced

Sad/low energy

Afternoon:

Great/energized

Neutral/balanced

Sad/low energy

Evening:

Great/energized

Neutral/balanced

Sad/low energy

How much/what type of exercise?

Personal Journal space

Doodle space

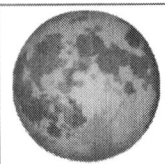

Phase of the moon

New   Waxing   Waning   Full

Date:

How I slept:

What I Ate:

Morning

_____
_____
_____

Afternoon

_____
_____
_____

Evening

_____
_____
_____

How I felt:

Morning:

Great/energized

Neutral/balanced

Sad/low energy

Afternoon:

Great/energized

Neutral/balanced

Sad/low energy

Evening:

Great/energized

Neutral/balanced

Sad/low energy

How much/what type of exercise?

Personal Journal space

Doodle space

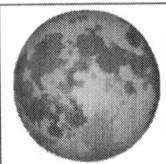 Phase of the moon New Waxing Waning Full	Date:

How I slept:

What I Ate:

Morning

_____

_____

_____

Afternoon

_____

_____

_____

Evening

_____

_____

_____

How much/what type of exercise?

How I felt:

Morning:

Great/energized

Neutral/balanced

Sad/low energy

Afternoon:

Great/energized

Neutral/balanced

Sad/low energy

Evening:

Great/energized

Neutral/balanced

Sad/low energy

Personal Journal space

Doodle space

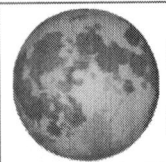

Phase of the moon

New   Waxing   Waning   Full

Date:

How I slept:

What I Ate:

Morning

_____

_____

_____

Afternoon

_____

_____

_____

Evening

_____

_____

_____

How I felt:

Morning:

Great/energized

Neutral/balanced

Sad/low energy

Afternoon:

Great/energized

Neutral/balanced

Sad/low energy

Evening:

Great/energized

Neutral/balanced

Sad/low energy

How much/what type of exercise?

Personal Journal space

Doodle space

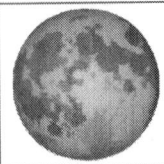 Phase of the moon

New   Waxing   Waning   Full

Date:

How I slept:

What I Ate:
  Morning

  _____
  _____
  _____

  Afternoon

  _____
  _____
  _____

  Evening

  _____
  _____
  _____

How I felt:

  Morning:

  Great/energized

  Neutral/balanced

  Sad/low energy

  Afternoon:

  Great/energized

  Neutral/balanced

  Sad/low energy

  Evening:

  Great/energized

  Neutral/balanced

  Sad/low energy

How much/what type of exercise?

Personal Journal space

Doodle space

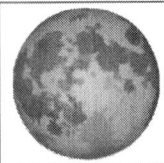 Phase of the moon

New   Waxing   Waning   Full

Date:

How I slept:

What I Ate:
   Morning

_____
_____
_____
_____

   Afternoon

_____
_____
_____
_____

   Evening

_____
_____
_____
_____

How I felt:

   Morning:

   Great/energized

   Neutral/balanced

   Sad/low energy

   Afternoon:

   Great/energized

   Neutral/balanced

   Sad/low energy

   Evening:

   Great/energized

   Neutral/balanced

   Sad/low energy

How much/what type of exercise?

Personal Journal space

Doodle space

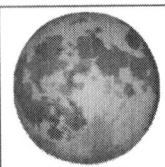

Phase of the moon

New   Waxing   Waning   Full

Date:

How I slept:

What I Ate:

Morning

_____
_____
_____

Afternoon

_____
_____
_____

Evening

_____
_____
_____

How I felt:

Morning:

Great/energized

Neutral/balanced

Sad/low energy

Afternoon:

Great/energized

Neutral/balanced

Sad/low energy

Evening:

Great/energized

Neutral/balanced

Sad/low energy

How much/what type of exercise?

Personal Journal space

Doodle space

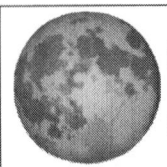

Phase of the moon

New   Waxing   Waning   Full

Date:

How I slept:

What I Ate:
   Morning

_____
_____
_____
_____

   Afternoon

_____
_____
_____
_____

   Evening

_____
_____
_____
_____

How I felt:
   Morning:

   Great/energized

   Neutral/balanced

   Sad/low energy

   Afternoon:

   Great/energized

   Neutral/balanced

   Sad/low energy

   Evening:

   Great/energized

   Neutral/balanced

   Sad/low energy

How much/what type of exercise?

Personal Journal space

Doodle space

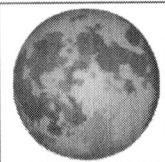 Phase of the moon

New   Waxing   Waning   Full

Date:

How I slept:

What I Ate:
 Morning

_____
_____
_____

 Afternoon

_____
_____
_____

 Evening

_____
_____
_____

How I felt:
 Morning:
  Great/energized
  Neutral/balanced
  Sad/low energy

 Afternoon:
  Great/energized
  Neutral/balanced
  Sad/low energy

 Evening:
  Great/energized
  Neutral/balanced
  Sad/low energy

How much/what type of exercise?

Personal Journal space

Doodle space

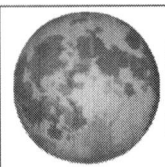

Phase of the moon

New   Waxing   Waning   Full

Date:

How I slept:

What I Ate:
　Morning

_____
_____
_____

　Afternoon

_____
_____
_____

　Evening

_____
_____
_____

How I felt:

　Morning:

　Great/energized

　Neutral/balanced

　Sad/low energy

　Afternoon:

　Great/energized

　Neutral/balanced

　Sad/low energy

　Evening:

　Great/energized

　Neutral/balanced

　Sad/low energy

How much/what type of exercise?

Personal Journal space

Doodle space

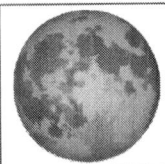 Phase of the moon

New   Waxing   Waning   Full

Date:

How I slept:

What I Ate:
 Morning

_____
_____
_____

 Afternoon

_____
_____
_____

 Evening

_____
_____
_____

How I felt:
 Morning:
  Great/energized
  Neutral/balanced
  Sad/low energy

 Afternoon:
  Great/energized
  Neutral/balanced
  Sad/low energy

 Evening:
  Great/energized
  Neutral/balanced
  Sad/low energy

How much/what type of exercise?

Personal Journal space

Doodle space

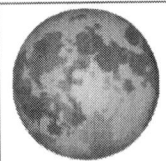

Phase of the moon

New Waxing Waning Full

Date:

How I slept:

What I Ate:

Morning

_____
_____
_____

Afternoon

_____
_____
_____

Evening

_____
_____
_____

How much/what type of exercise?

How I felt:

Morning:

Great/energized

Neutral/balanced

Sad/low energy

Afternoon:

Great/energized

Neutral/balanced

Sad/low energy

Evening:

Great/energized

Neutral/balanced

Sad/low energy

Personal Journal space

Doodle space

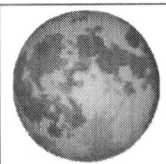 Phase of the moon New Waxing Waning Full	Date:

How I slept:

What I Ate:

Morning

_____
_____
_____

Afternoon

_____
_____
_____

Evening

_____
_____
_____

How I felt:

Morning:

Great/energized

Neutral/balanced

Sad/low energy

Afternoon:

Great/energized

Neutral/balanced

Sad/low energy

Evening:

Great/energized

Neutral/balanced

Sad/low energy

How much/what type of exercise?

Personal Journal space

Doodle space

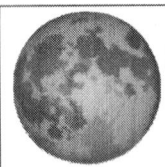 Phase of the moon New Waxing Waning Full	Date:

How I slept:

What I Ate:

Morning

_____
_____
_____

Afternoon

_____
_____
_____

Evening

_____
_____
_____

How I felt:

Morning:

Great/energized

Neutral/balanced

Sad/low energy

Afternoon:

Great/energized

Neutral/balanced

Sad/low energy

Evening:

Great/energized

Neutral/balanced

Sad/low energy

How much/what type of exercise?

Personal Journal space

Doodle space

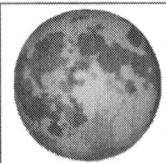 Phase of the moon

New   Waxing   Waning   Full

Date:

How I slept:

What I Ate:
　Morning

_____
_____
_____

　Afternoon

_____
_____
_____

　Evening

_____
_____
_____

How I felt:

　Morning:

　　Great/energized

　　Neutral/balanced

　　Sad/low energy

　Afternoon:

　　Great/energized

　　Neutral/balanced

　　Sad/low energy

　Evening:

　　Great/energized

　　Neutral/balanced

　　Sad/low energy

How much/what type of exercise?

Personal Journal space

Doodle space

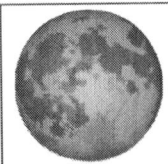 Phase of the moon

New   Waxing   Waning   Full

Date:

How I slept:

What I Ate:

Morning

_____
_____
_____
_____

Afternoon

_____
_____
_____
_____

Evening

_____
_____
_____
_____

How I felt:

Morning:

Great/energized

Neutral/balanced

Sad/low energy

Afternoon:

Great/energized

Neutral/balanced

Sad/low energy

Evening:

Great/energized

Neutral/balanced

Sad/low energy

How much/what type of exercise?

Personal Journal space

Doodle space

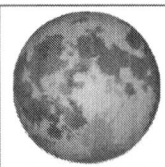 Phase of the moon New Waxing Waning Full	Date:

How I slept:

What I Ate:
   Morning

_____
_____
_____

   Afternoon

_____
_____
_____

   Evening

_____
_____
_____

How I felt:
   Morning:
      Great/energized
      Neutral/balanced
      Sad/low energy

   Afternoon:
      Great/energized
      Neutral/balanced
      Sad/low energy

   Evening:
      Great/energized
      Neutral/balanced
      Sad/low energy

How much/what type of exercise?

Personal Journal space

Doodle space

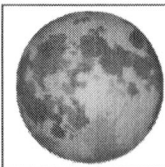 Phase of the moon

New   Waxing   Waning   Full

Date:

How I slept:

What I Ate:
   Morning

_____
_____
_____

   Afternoon

_____
_____
_____

   Evening

_____
_____
_____

How I felt:
   Morning:
      Great/energized
      Neutral/balanced
      Sad/low energy

   Afternoon:
      Great/energized
      Neutral/balanced
      Sad/low energy

   Evening:
      Great/energized
      Neutral/balanced
      Sad/low energy

How much/what type of exercise?

Personal Journal space

Doodle space

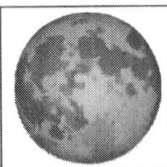 Phase of the moon

New   Waxing   Waning   Full

Date:

How I slept:

What I Ate:
Morning

_____
_____
_____

Afternoon

_____
_____
_____

Evening

_____
_____
_____

How I felt:

Morning:

Great/energized

Neutral/balanced

Sad/low energy

Afternoon:

Great/energized

Neutral/balanced

Sad/low energy

Evening:

Great/energized

Neutral/balanced

Sad/low energy

How much/what type of exercise?

Personal Journal space

Doodle space

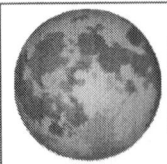 Phase of the moon

New   Waxing   Waning   Full

Date:

How I slept:

What I Ate:

Morning

_____
_____
_____
_____

Afternoon

_____
_____
_____
_____

Evening

_____
_____
_____
_____

How I felt:

Morning:

Great/energized

Neutral/balanced

Sad/low energy

Afternoon:

Great/energized

Neutral/balanced

Sad/low energy

Evening:

Great/energized

Neutral/balanced

Sad/low energy

How much/what type of exercise?

Personal Journal space

Doodle space

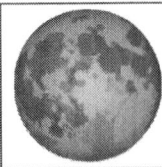 Phase of the moon

New   Waxing   Waning   Full

Date:

How I slept:

What I Ate:
Morning

How I felt:
Morning:

Great/energized

Neutral/balanced

Sad/low energy

Afternoon

Afternoon:

Great/energized

Neutral/balanced

Sad/low energy

Evening

Evening:

Great/energized

Neutral/balanced

Sad/low energy

How much/what type of exercise?

Personal Journal space

Doodle space

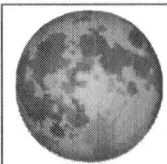

Phase of the moon

New   Waxing   Waning   Full

Date:

How I slept:

What I Ate:
 Morning

How I felt:
 Morning:
  Great/energized
  Neutral/balanced
  Sad/low energy

 Afternoon

 Afternoon:
  Great/energized
  Neutral/balanced
  Sad/low energy

 Evening

 Evening:
  Great/energized
  Neutral/balanced
  Sad/low energy

How much/what type of exercise?

Personal Journal space

Doodle space

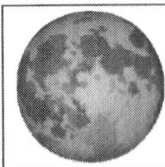 Phase of the moon

New   Waxing   Waning   Full

Date:

How I slept:

What I Ate:
   Morning

_____
_____
_____

   Afternoon

_____
_____
_____

   Evening

_____
_____
_____

How I felt:
   Morning:

   Great/energized

   Neutral/balanced

   Sad/low energy

   Afternoon:

   Great/energized

   Neutral/balanced

   Sad/low energy

   Evening:

   Great/energized

   Neutral/balanced

   Sad/low energy

How much/what type of exercise?

Personal Journal space

Doodle space

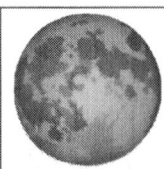 Phase of the moon

New   Waxing   Waning   Full

Date:

How I slept:

What I Ate:
  Morning
  _____
  _____
  _____

  Afternoon
  _____
  _____
  _____

  Evening
  _____
  _____
  _____

How I felt:
  Morning:
    Great/energized
    Neutral/balanced
    Sad/low energy

  Afternoon:
    Great/energized
    Neutral/balanced
    Sad/low energy

  Evening:
    Great/energized
    Neutral/balanced
    Sad/low energy

How much/what type of exercise?

Personal Journal space

Doodle space

2017-18 Phases of the moon

2017

New Moon	Full Moon
28-Jan	12-Jan
26-Feb	11-Feb
28-Mar	12-Mar
26-Apr	11-Apr
25-May	10-May
24-Jun	9-Jun
23-Jul	9-Jul
21-Aug	7-Aug
20-Sep	6-Sep
19-Oct	5-Oct
18-Nov	4-Nov
18-Dec	3-Dec

2018

New Moon	Full Moon
16-Jan	31-Jan
15-Feb	1-Mar
17-Mar	31-Mar
15-Apr	29-Apr
15-May	29-May
13-Jun	28-Jun
12-Jul	27-Jul
11-Aug	26-Aug
9-Sep	24-Sep
8-Oct	24-Oct
7-Nov	23-Nov
7-Dec	22-Dec

Source: https://www.timeanddate.com/moon/phases

Made in the USA
Middletown, DE
19 December 2017